MICHAEL C. GILBERT

WHAT YOUR DOCTOR MAY NOT TELL YOU ABOUT PEPTIC ULCERS

A JOURNEY TO UNDERSTANDING, EMPOWERING, AND CONQUERING STOMACH ULCERS

First Edition

Advisor: TIMOTHY E. FREEMAN

Advisor: LEONARD P. DICKERSON

Advisor: DR. LEWIS PAGE

Advisor: DR. VICTORIA O'NEILL

Preface

Welcome to the pages of "What Your Doctor May Not Tell You About Peptic Ulcers." The goal of writing this book is to help people who are dealing with peptic ulcers and want more than just medical advice—it's a holistic view of their path to health.

In these sections, we leave on a complete investigation, unwinding the complexities of peptic ulcers and offering an aid intended for the people who might be experiencing this well being challenge. Whether you're looking for lucidity about side effects, digging into counteraction techniques, or exploring the subtleties of long-term well being support, this book is a friend as you continue looking for stomach-related health.

The excursion through these pages is definitely not a singular one. It's an aggregate endeavor—a discourse between the information refined inside these words and the special encounters every peruse brings. From understanding the causes and side effects to dispersing fantasies and tending to normal worries, each part is a venturing stone toward a more educated and versatile way to deal with peptic ulcers.

As you dive into the parts, think about this book as a wellspring of data as well as a sidekick on your way to prosperity. Embrace the strengthening that accompanies information, and use it to team up with medical services experts, pursue informed decisions, and develop a way of life that upholds your stomach-related well being.

Peptic ulcers might introduce difficulties, yet inside those difficulties lie open doors for development, flexibility, and a recharged obligation to your prosperity. Allow this book to be your aide, your partner, and your wellspring of lucidity on the excursion to understanding and overseeing peptic ulcers.

May these words illuminate the way to digestive health and serve as a beacon of knowledge.

Warm respects,

MICHAEL C. GILBERT

Acknowledgement

The notion that every creative work is a collective effort comes into clear focus when bringing "What Your Doctor May Not Tell You About Peptic Ulcers" to completion. I want to express my deepest thanks to everyone who has helped and contributed to this adventure.

Your knowledge and devotion form the core of this effort for the committed healthcare professionals who work diligently to improve the lives of those afflicted by peptic ulcers. Your continuous commitment to patient care is an inspiration.

Your unwavering support has been the foundation of my resilience, friends and family, whose encouragement gave the essential fire for my attempt. Your empathy during times of solitude and your joyous attitude around anniversaries are treasured beyond words.

May the lessons contained within these pages serve as a light of wisdom to all who begin on this journey, providing clarity and empowerment in the face of health issues.

This book is a tapestry made from the threads of communal work, and each individual named here had an important part in its development. Thank you for joining us on this journey toward greater knowledge, resilience, and well-being.

With heartfelt gratitude,

MICHAEL C. GILBERT

TABLE OF CONTENTS

1

INTRODUCTION

UNDERSTANDING PEPTIC ULCERS

Peptic ulcers are a prevalent but generally mistaken sickness that might substantially affect a person's own happiness. We hope to explain and empower readers who may be coping with this gastrointestinal ailment by going into the principles of peptic ulcers in this initial chapter. This chapter offers a starting point for those who have peptic ulcers and wish to learn how to better manage their illness.

At its heart, a peptic ulcer is an open sore that forms on the inward coating of the stomach, small digestive system, or throat. The stomach's digestive juices and the processes that protect the lining from their corrosive effects are out of balance, generating these ulcers. Understanding the concept of these ulcers is vital for individuals battling with the condition, as it shapes the cause for educated navigation and strong administration.

Peptic ulcers arrive in numerous types, with the most commonly known being gastric ulcers that develop in the stomach and duodenal ulcers that form in the upper component of the small digestive system. Understanding the intricacies of these signs is vital for fast diagnosis and treatment, despite the fact that the symptoms might range from scorching stomach pain to nausea and bloating. In order to give readers a full grasp of what to look for and when to seek medical assistance, the purpose of this chapter is to simplify these symptoms.

The causes and chance aspects leading to peptic ulcers are multi-layered. From bacterial sickness, typically linked with Helicobacter pylori, to the far-reaching use of non steroidal mitigating medicines (NSAIDs), the pathogenesis of peptic ulcers contains a complex combination of factors.

By disentangling these providers, individuals may all the more likely apprehend the origins of their issue, working with extra-informed chats with medical care specialists.

The expedition of knowing peptic ulcers incorporates recognizing the analytic cycles and clinical trials employed by medical services providers. Sections to follow will dig more into these tactics, but this beginning section takes a fast look into the importance of teaming up with healthcare specialists to detect and understand the notion of one's ulcer.

Generally, this part fills in as a gateway to full research on peptic ulcers. It urges readers to go on a path of self-knowledge and self-discovery, providing an environment in which people with this disease may conquer barriers with confidence and understanding. The objective of this book isn't just to train, but also to engage folks to successfully take part in their medical care venture, provided with the pieces of information necessary to come to informed judgments regarding their peptic ulcer.

IMPORTANCE OF KNOWLEDGE FOR PATIENTS

In the domain of medical care, information is obviously an amazing asset, and for patients managing peptic ulcers, it turns into a foundation for viable administration and works towards prosperity. Understanding the meaning of obtaining information about one's condition is fundamental, as it enables people to effectively partake in their medical care venture, pursue informed choices, and cultivate a cooperative relationship with medical services experts.

Knowledge, first and foremost, is a catalyst for prompt intervention and early detection. People are better able to identify potential problems with their gastrointestinal health when they are aware of the symptoms that are associated with peptic ulcers. This early mindfulness can incite opportune clinical interviews, prompting swifter determinations and more powerful treatment procedures. The maxim "information is power" rings especially obvious with regards to medical care, where informed patients are better situated to advocate for their prosperity.

In addition, an educated patient is better prepared to participate in significant conversations with medical service suppliers. Equipped with information about peptic ulcers, people can effectively partake in their treatment plans, pose relevant inquiries, and fathom the reasoning behind endorsed medications and way of life suggestions. This cooperative methodology among patients and medical services experts encourages a feeling of organization and shared understanding, establishing a more steady medical services climate.

The significance of information reaches out past the domains of finding and treatment. It assumes a significant part in directing way of life changes and preventive measures. With a complete comprehension of elements that add to peptic ulcers, for example, dietary decisions and stress the executives, patients can pursue educated choices to decrease the probability regarding repeat and advance long haul stomach related well being.

Moreover, mindfulness enables patients to address normal misinterpretations and legends encompassing peptic ulcers. People can avoid unnecessary anxiety and adopt evidence-based approaches to their health by dispelling false information and making decisions based on accurate information.

Generally, the significance of information for patients managing peptic ulcers couldn't possibly be more significant. It frames the bedrock for proactive medical services commitment, empowering people to explore their clinical excursion with certainty and versatility. As we dig into the complexities of peptic ulcers in ensuing sections, the all-encompassing objective is to outfit perusers with the information important to pursue informed decisions, advocate for their prosperity, and eventually improve their personal satisfaction.

2

THE ANATOMY OF STOMACH AND DUODENUM

The anatomy of the stomach and duodenum is a complex interplay of structures and functions crucial to the digestive process. The stomach, situated immediately distal to the esophagus, consists of distinct regions: the cardia, the upper fundus located beneath the left diaphragm, the mid-region or body, and the antrum extending to the pylorus. Functioning as a reservoir, the stomach retains and breaks down food before actively expelling it into the proximal small intestine.

The smooth muscle of the stomach wall exhibits three layers: outer longitudinal, inner circular, and innermost oblique layers. Two sphincters, the gastro-esophageal sphincter and the pyloric sphincter, regulate the flow of gastric contents. The pyloric sphincter, primarily composed of a thickening of the circular muscle layer, controls the exit of gastric contents into the duodenum.

Moving into the duodenum, it possesses outer longitudinal and inner circular smooth muscle layers. The duodenum, shaped like a 'C,' accommodates the pancreas within its concavity and terminates at the duodenojejunal flexure, where it connects to the jejunum.

The mucosal lining of the stomach is dynamic, capable of stretching with feeding. The greater curvature of the undistended stomach features thick folds or rugae. In the upper two-thirds of the stomach's mucosa, parietal cells secrete hydrochloric acid, while chief cells secrete pepsinogen, initiating proteolysis. A noticeable color change often occurs at the junction between the stomach's body and antrum, visible macroscopically and confirmed by measuring surface pH.

Within the antral mucosa, bicarbonate secretion and the presence of mucus-secreting cells and G cells, which stimulate acid production, contribute to the digestive process. Gastrin, in two major forms (G17 and G34), plays a crucial role in this process. Somatostatin, produced by specialized antral cells (D cells), acts as a suppressant of acid secretion.

Throughout the stomach, mucus-secreting cells are present, contributing to the production of mucus and bicarbonate. The mucus itself consists of glycoproteins called mucins. The 'Mucosal Barrier,' formed by the plasma membranes of mucosal cells and the mucus layer, acts as a protective shield for the gastric epithelium. This barrier shields against damage caused by acid, alcohol, aspirin, non-steroidal anti-inflammatory drugs (NSAIDs), and bile salts. Prostaglandins stimulate mucus secretion, and their synthesis is inhibited by aspirin and NSAIDs, which target cyclo-oxygenase.

Transitioning to the duodenum, its mucosa features villi, akin to the rest of the small bowel, and includes Brunner's glands that secrete alkaline mucus. This, in conjunction with pancreatic and biliary secretions, aids in neutralizing the acidic content from the stomach upon reaching the duodenum.

The intricate anatomy of the stomach and duodenum orchestrates a symphony of physiological processes essential for digestion and nutrient absorption. From the muscular layers to the diverse cell types and the protective mucosal barrier, each component contributes to the seamless functioning of the gastrointestinal system. Understanding these intricacies provides valuable insights into digestive health and the mechanisms underlying various gastrointestinal conditions.

THE PHYSIOLOGY

In the intricate physiology of the stomach, acid secretion plays a pivotal role, not only in digestion but also as a defense mechanism against certain food-borne infections. This process is finely regulated by both neural and hormonal influences. Histamine, directly acting on parietal cells, is stimulated by acetylcholine and gastrin, released via enterochromaffin cells.

However, the intricate balance is maintained by somatostatin, which inhibits both histamine and gastrin release, thereby regulating acid secretion. Beyond acid secretion, the stomach serves multiple vital functions, acting as a reservoir for food, facilitating emulsification of fats, mixing gastric contents, and secreting intrinsic factors crucial for absorption

. The intricacies of gastric emptying involve factors such as osmoreceptors in the duodenal mucosa, orchestrating local reflexes and the release of gut hormones.

Notably, intraduodenal fat introduces negative feedback, causing a delay in gastric emptying through duodenal receptors, revealing the complexity of the digestive orchestration within the gastrointestinal system.

3

WHAT IS A PEPTIC ULCER?

A peptic ulcer is a chronic, open sore that forms on the inner lining of the stomach, upper small intestine (duodenum), or, less commonly, the esophagus. These ulcers develop when the protective layer of mucus that usually guards the digestive tract is compromised, allowing stomach acids to erode the sensitive lining beneath.

DEFINITION:

Peptic ulcers typically arise from an imbalance between aggressive factors like stomach acid and digestive enzymes, and the protective mechanisms that shield the gastrointestinal lining. The primary culprits often include Helicobacter pylori (H. pylori) infection and the use of nonsteroidal anti-inflammatory drugs (NSAIDs), both of which can weaken the mucosal defenses.

Understanding the dynamics of a peptic ulcer involves recognizing its chronic nature. Unlike superficial wounds, these ulcers persist over time, requiring targeted medical attention for proper management.

TYPES

1. GASTRIC ULCERS

- Located in the stomach lining.
- Symptoms may include burning stomach pain, bloating, and nausea.

2. DUODENAL ULCERS

- Form in the upper part of the small intestine (duodenum).
- Often characterized by a burning or gnawing pain in the abdomen, occurring between meals or during the night.

3. ESOPHAGEAL ULCERS

- Less common but can occur in the lower part of the esophagus.
- Associated with symptoms like difficulty swallowing and chest pain.

4. STRESS ULCERS

- Linked to severe physical trauma, injury, or critical illness.
- Tend to affect the stomach lining and can be more acute.

5. REFRACTORY ULCERS

- Occur when standard treatments are ineffective.
- May necessitate more advanced therapies and closer monitoring.

Each type of peptic ulcer presents its own set of symptoms and challenges, making accurate diagnosis crucial for tailored treatment. While some individuals may experience discomfort and pain, others may remain asymptomatic, underscoring the importance of medical evaluation for a comprehensive understanding of the condition.

As we explore peptic ulcers further in subsequent chapters, the goal is to provide insights into effective management strategies, empowering individuals to navigate the complexities of their condition with knowledge and confidence.

CAUSES AND RISK FACTORS OF PEPTIC ULCERS

Peptic ulcers, though common, often result from a complex interplay of various factors. Understanding the causes and risk factors behind these gastric sores is crucial for both prevention and effective management.

HELICOBACTER PYLORI (H. PYLORI) INFECTION:

One of the primary causes of peptic ulcers is infection with Helicobacter pylori bacteria. This microorganism can weaken the protective mucus layer in the stomach and duodenum, making the lining more susceptible to the corrosive effects of stomach acid. H. pylori is a common infection, and its presence does not always lead to ulcers, but it is a significant risk factor.

NONSTEROIDAL ANTI-INFLAMMATORY DRUGS (NSAIDS):

Regular use of NSAIDs, such as aspirin, ibuprofen, and naproxen, can increase the risk of peptic ulcers. These medications can irritate the stomach lining and compromise the protective mechanisms, making it easier for ulcers to develop. Individuals using NSAIDs regularly, especially in high doses or over extended periods, should be cautious and consider preventive measures.

ACID OVERPRODUCTION:

In some cases, overproduction of stomach acid can contribute to the development of peptic ulcers. Conditions like Zollinger-Ellison syndrome, a rare tumor that increases acid production, can elevate the risk. Understanding and managing conditions associated with excessive acid secretion is essential in these cases.

SMOKING AND ALCOHOL CONSUMPTION:

Smoking and excessive alcohol consumption are lifestyle factors that can heighten the risk of peptic ulcers. Both habits can irritate the stomach lining and compromise its integrity. Quitting smoking and moderating alcohol intake can be beneficial in preventing ulcer formation and promoting overall digestive health.

AGE AND GENETICS:

While peptic ulcers can affect individuals of any age, older adults may be more susceptible. Additionally, there is evidence of a genetic predisposition to peptic ulcers. A family history of ulcers or related conditions may increase an individual's risk.

STRESS AND DIET:

While stress itself is not a direct cause of peptic ulcers, it can exacerbate existing conditions. Poor stress management may lead to unhealthy lifestyle choices, such as a diet high in spicy foods, which can contribute to ulcer development. Adopting stress-reduction techniques and maintaining a balanced diet are integral aspects of prevention.

Understanding these causes and risk factors is pivotal to adopting preventive measures and seeking timely medical attention when necessary. In the subsequent chapters, we'll delve deeper into diagnostic processes, treatment options, and lifestyle modifications to empower individuals to manage and mitigate the impact of peptic ulcers on their health.

4

HELICOBACTER PYLORI

Helicobacter pylori is a distinctive, slow-growing, spiral-shaped bacterium with a Gram-negative nature and flagella. It possesses the unique ability to produce urease, a key factor in its involvement in gastritis and the development of peptic ulcer disease. This bacterium establishes residence within the mucous layer of the gastric antrum, and intriguingly, it also inhabits areas of gastric metaplasia in the duodenum. Within the gastric pits, H. pylori exhibits a specific affinity for gastric epithelial cells, positioning itself in higher concentrations under the protective mucous layer. Notably, this layer serves as a shield against gastric acid, and its effectiveness is augmented by the retention of bicarbonate secreted by antral cells and the ammonia produced through bacterial urease activity.

EPIDEMIOLOGY

Epidemiological trends reveal a stark contrast in the prevalence of H. pylori, with developing countries exhibiting high rates (80–90% of the population) and developed countries experiencing a lower prevalence (20–50%). Notably, infection rates are notably elevated in lower-income demographics.

The acquisition of H. pylori typically occurs during childhood, and while the exact transmission route remains uncertain, possibilities include fecal-oral or oral-oral pathways. Intriguingly, the incidence of infection rises with age, likely linked to childhood acquisition during periods of lower hygiene standards, rather than adult-onset infections, which are significantly less common, accounting for far less than 1% per year in developed countries.

PATHOGENESIS

While the intricate mechanisms driving pathogenesis remain partially elusive, a significant portion of the colonized population experiences lifelong asymptomatic colonization. Helicobacter pylori displays remarkable adaptability to the stomach environment, selectively residing in the gastric epithelium and positioning itself within or just beneath the protective mucous layer.

The adherence of H. pylori relies on various adhesion molecules, including BabA, forming bonds with the Lewis antigen present on the surface of gastric mucosal cells. This interaction triggers gastritis in all infected individuals. The pathogen inflicts damage to gastric epithelial cells by releasing enzymes and inducing apoptosis through binding to class I major histocompatibility complex (MHC) molecules.

Critical to its pathogenicity, H. pylori's urease production facilitates the conversion of urea into ammonium and chloride, exerting direct cytotoxic effects. Notably, the prevalence of ulcers is most pronounced when the infecting strain expresses the CagA (cytotoxic-associated protein) and VacA (vacuolating toxin) genes. This expression intensifies the inflammatory and immune response, leading to a higher likelihood of ulcer formation. The CagA and VacA genes are correlated with increased interleukin 8 (IL-8) induction, a potent mediator of gastric inflammation.

Furthermore, the host's genetic makeup plays a role in this intricate interplay. Genetic variations, such as polymorphisms that elevate IL-1β levels, are associated with atrophic gastritis and an increased risk of developing cancer. This multifaceted interaction between H. pylori's virulence factors and the host's genetic variations contributes to the diverse clinical outcomes observed in individuals infected with this bacterium.

5

COMMON SIGNS AND INDICATORS OF PEPTIC ULCERS

Recognizing the signs and indicators of peptic ulcers is crucial for early detection and prompt intervention. While symptoms may vary among individuals, understanding the common signals associated with these gastric sores can empower individuals to seek timely medical attention and initiate effective management strategies.

1. BURNING ABDOMINAL PAIN:

A hallmark symptom of peptic ulcers is a persistent burning or gnawing pain in the upper abdomen. This discomfort may be felt between meals, during the night, or when the stomach is empty.

2. HEARTBURN OR INDIGESTION:

Individuals with peptic ulcers may experience frequent heartburn or indigestion. This sensation is often described as a burning feeling in the chest or throat and can occur shortly after eating.

3. NAUSEA AND VOMITING:

Peptic ulcers can lead to feelings of nausea, which may occasionally progress to vomiting. Persistent or severe nausea should prompt a medical evaluation.

4. CHANGES IN APPETITE AND WEIGHT LOSS:

Some individuals with peptic ulcers may experience changes in appetite, ranging from a decreased desire to eat to early satiety. Unintentional weight loss may also be observed.

5. BLOATING AND FULLNESS:

Bloating and a sense of fullness, even after consuming small amounts of food, can be indicative of peptic ulcers. These symptoms may be more pronounced in the upper abdomen.

6. BLOOD IN STOOL OR VOMIT:

In more severe cases, peptic ulcers can lead to gastrointestinal bleeding. This may manifest as blood in the stool, which can appear dark and tarry, or in vomit, which presents as coffee-ground-like material.

7. DIFFICULTY SWALLOWING:

Esophageal ulcers, although less common, may cause difficulty swallowing. This symptom requires prompt medical attention for further evaluation.

It's important to note that some individuals with peptic ulcers may remain asymptomatic, especially during the early stages. Regular medical check-ups and attention to any unusual digestive symptoms can aid in early detection and effective management.

If you are experiencing persistent or worsening symptoms associated with peptic ulcers, seeking consultation with a healthcare professional is crucial. Diagnostic procedures, such as endoscopy and imaging tests, can provide a definitive diagnosis, allowing for targeted and personalized treatment approaches. As we delve into subsequent chapters, we'll explore these diagnostic methods and delve deeper into effective strategies for managing peptic ulcers.

CLINICAL MANIFESTATIONS OF PEPTIC ULCER DISEASE

A distinctive hallmark of peptic ulcer disease is the recurring, burning epigastric pain. Research indicates that when a patient points to the epigastrium with a single finger, strongly indicating the location of the pain, it is a notable sign of potential peptic ulcer disease. The connection between pain and food intake varies and, overall, does not significantly aid in diagnosis.

In duodenal ulcers (DUs), the pain classically occurs at night, more intensely when the patient is hungry; however, this pattern is not consistently reliable. Gastric ulcers (GUs) and DUs alike may find relief through the use of antacids. Nausea may accompany the pain, and though vomiting is infrequent, it can provide relief. Anorexia and weight loss may be more pronounced in cases of GUs. Persistent and severe pain may indicate complications, such as penetration into adjacent organs. Back pain may suggest the presence of a penetrating posterior ulcer. Interestingly, severe ulceration can sometimes manifest without noticeable symptoms, as individuals presenting with acute ulcer bleeding or perforation may not have experienced preceding ulcer-related symptoms.

In the absence of intervention, the symptoms of a duodenal ulcer may exhibit spontaneous relapses and remissions. The natural progression of the disease involves a gradual remission over several years, attributed to the onset of atrophic gastritis and a decline in acid secretion. This unique trajectory underscores the variable and nuanced nature of peptic ulcer disease clinical manifestations.

WHEN TO SEEK MEDICAL ATTENTION FOR PEPTIC ULCERS

Knowing when to seek medical attention is paramount for individuals experiencing symptoms or concerned about the possibility of peptic ulcers. While some symptoms may be mild and intermittent, others could indicate more serious complications. Here are guidelines on when to promptly consult with a healthcare professional:

1. PERSISTENT ABDOMINAL PAIN:

If you experience persistent, recurrent abdominal pain, especially a burning or gnawing sensation in the upper abdomen, it's essential to seek medical attention. This pain may not always be severe but should be evaluated, especially if it disrupts your daily activities.

2. SIGNIFICANT CHANGES IN DIGESTIVE PATTERNS:

Any significant changes in digestive patterns, such as persistent heartburn, indigestion, nausea, or vomiting, should prompt a visit to a healthcare provider. These symptoms may be indicative of underlying issues, including peptic ulcers.

3. UNEXPLAINED WEIGHT LOSS:

If you are experiencing unintentional weight loss without changes in diet or physical activity, it could be a sign of a more advanced condition. Consultation with a healthcare professional is crucial to identifying the underlying cause.

4. BLOOD IN STOOL OR VOMIT:

The presence of blood in stool, which may appear dark and tarry, or in vomit (resembling coffee grounds) is a serious symptom that requires immediate medical attention. This may indicate gastrointestinal bleeding associated with peptic ulcers.

5. DIFFICULTY SWALLOWING:

Difficulty swallowing, particularly if accompanied by pain or discomfort, may suggest complications such as esophageal ulcers. Seeking medical advice promptly is essential for a thorough evaluation.

6. PERSISTENT FATIGUE OR WEAKNESS:

Chronic fatigue or weakness, often unrelated to exertion or lack of sleep, may be associated with anemia resulting from peptic ulcer-related bleeding. This requires a prompt medical assessment.

7. WORSENING SYMPTOMS DESPITE LIFESTYLE CHANGES:

If you've implemented lifestyle modifications recommended for managing peptic ulcers but notice worsening symptoms or no improvement, it's crucial to consult with a healthcare professional for a comprehensive evaluation.

8. HISTORY OF NSAID OR ASPIRIN USE:

Individuals with a history of regular NSAID or aspirin use should be vigilant about monitoring for peptic ulcer symptoms. If any signs emerge, seeking medical attention early on can prevent complications.

Remember, early detection and intervention contribute significantly to successful peptic ulcer management. If in doubt or experiencing persistent symptoms, consulting with a healthcare provider is the prudent course of action. Diagnostic tests, such as endoscopy and imaging, can provide a clear understanding of the underlying issues, facilitating the development of an appropriate treatment plan. In the subsequent chapters, we'll explore various aspects of diagnosis, treatment, and preventive measures to empower individuals to effectively manage peptic ulcers.

6

DIAGNOSIS AND MEDICAL TESTS

PROCEDURES FOR IDENTIFYING PEPTIC ULCERS

Embarking on the journey of identifying peptic ulcers involves a series of diagnostic procedures aimed at unraveling the complexities of this gastrointestinal condition. The process integrates a range of medical tests, each contributing a unique perspective to the comprehensive understanding of peptic ulcers.

1. CLINICAL ASSESSMENT:

The initial step involves a thorough clinical assessment, where healthcare professionals delve into the patient's medical history, symptoms, and lifestyle factors. This holistic approach lays the groundwork for more targeted diagnostic investigations.

2. ENDOSCOPY:

Utilizing advanced technology, endoscopy offers a direct visual examination of the upper gastrointestinal tract. A flexible tube with a camera allows clinicians to inspect the lining of the esophagus, stomach, and duodenum. This procedure is instrumental in identifying the presence of ulcers and assessing their characteristics.

3. UPPER GASTROINTESTINAL SERIES (UGI):

An upper gastrointestinal series involving the consumption of a contrast agent followed by X-ray imaging provides valuable insights into the structural integrity of the digestive organs. This aids in identifying abnormalities, including ulcers.

4. HELICOBACTER PYLORI TESTING:

Given the strong association between H. pylori infection and peptic ulcers, specific tests are conducted to detect the presence of this bacterium. These may include blood tests, stool tests, or breath tests that measure the byproducts of H. pylori metabolism.

5. CT scans or MRI:

In certain cases, computed tomography (CT) scans or magnetic resonance imaging (MRI) may be employed to assess the extent of complications or the penetration of ulcers into surrounding tissues.

6. BIOPSY:

Endoscopic procedures often involve taking tissue samples (biopsies) from suspicious areas. Analyzing these samples under a microscope helps confirm the presence of ulcers and determine if any cellular abnormalities are present.

7. LABORATORY TESTS:

Blood tests may be conducted to evaluate specific markers associated with peptic ulcers, such as levels of digestive enzymes or markers of inflammation.

Each diagnostic avenue contributes a unique facet to the overall diagnostic picture, allowing healthcare professionals to tailor treatment strategies to the individual needs of the patient. As we delve deeper into understanding peptic ulcers, these diagnostic insights become integral to crafting personalized and effective management plans.

Detecting Helicobacter pylori infection becomes imperative when considering treatment following a positive result. This typically occurs in scenarios involving active peptic ulcer disease, a history of peptic ulcer disease, or mucosa-associated lymphoid tissue (MALT) lymphoma. Additionally, the approach of 'test and treat' is applied to patients under 55 with dyspepsia and devoid of alarm symptoms, such as weight loss, anemia, dysphagia, vomiting, or a family history of gastrointestinal cancer. Clinical examination is often uninformative in these contexts.

FURTHER INVESTIGATIONS

EXPLORATION OF SUSPECTED PEPTIC ULCER DISEASE

Individuals below 55 years old displaying typical symptoms of peptic ulcer disease and testing positive for H. pylori can initiate eradication therapy without the need for additional investigations.

For older patients, a more thorough approach is essential, involving endoscopic diagnosis and the exclusion of cancer.

In cases of gastric ulcers, comprehensive biopsy procedures are imperative to rule out underlying malignancies, with follow-up endoscopic assessments until complete healing occurs.

Patients manifesting alarm symptoms necessitate endoscopy, encompassing:

- Iron deficiency anemia
- Weight loss
- Anorexia
- Hematemesis/melena
- Persistent vomiting
- Epigastric mass

This distinct approach ensures tailored investigations based on age, symptoms, and risk factors, providing a nuanced strategy for the diagnosis of suspected peptic ulcer disease.

COLLABORATING WITH HEALTHCARE PROFESSIONALS

Navigating the intricacies of health and well-being involves a collaborative partnership with healthcare professionals, an alliance geared towards understanding and addressing individual needs. This unique synergy forms the cornerstone of a personalized healthcare journey, where active engagement and communication empower both patients and healthcare providers.

1. OPEN DIALOGUE AND SHARED DECISION-MAKING:

Embrace an environment of open dialogue where your experiences, concerns, and questions find a receptive audience. Shared decision-making becomes a guiding principle, allowing you to actively participate in shaping your healthcare plan.

2. HOLISTIC UNDERSTANDING OF YOUR HEALTH:

Beyond specific symptoms, healthcare professionals strive for a holistic understanding of your health. This involves exploring lifestyle factors, emotional well-being, and unique circumstances, ensuring a comprehensive approach to your care.

3. INFORMED CHOICES AND EDUCATION:

As a partner in your healthcare, seek to be well-informed. Healthcare professionals are not just providers of care but educators, offering insights into conditions, treatments, and preventive measures. This knowledge empowers you to make informed choices aligned with your well-being.

4. TAILORED TREATMENT PLANS:

Recognize the uniqueness of your health journey. Working closely with healthcare professionals allows for the creation of tailored treatment plans that consider your individual needs, preferences, and lifestyle. This collaborative approach enhances the efficacy of interventions.

5. PROACTIVE HEALTH MANAGEMENT:

Shift from a reactive to a proactive approach to managing your health. Regular check-ins, preventive measures, and lifestyle adjustments become collaborative efforts, with healthcare professionals guiding and supporting your proactive health management.

6. CULTIVATING TRUST AND RAPPORT:

Trust is the bedrock of any effective healthcare collaboration. Cultivate a relationship built on mutual trust and rapport. This foundation fosters a sense of security, encouraging open communication and a shared commitment to your well-being.

In this distinctive partnership, you are not merely a recipient of care but an active participant in your health narrative. Embrace the opportunity to collaborate with healthcare professionals, recognizing the richness that arises when knowledge, experience, and personal insights converge to shape a healthcare journey uniquely tailored to you.

7

TREATMENT PATHWAYS

MEDICATIONS AND THEIR EFFECTS

Embarking on the road to recovery involves a nuanced exploration of treatment options, where medications play a pivotal role in shaping the trajectory of healing. This distinctive journey unfolds as medications weave their effects, tailored to address individual needs and foster a personalized approach to well-being.

1. PRECISION IN MEDICATION SELECTION:

The realm of treatment extends beyond a one-size-fits-all approach. Healthcare professionals, with a keen understanding of your health profile, carefully select medications tailored to your specific condition. This precision ensures that the therapeutic impact aligns seamlessly with your unique health requirements.

2. TARGETING THE ROOT CAUSE:

Medications act as strategic allies, targeting the root cause of your health challenges. Whether addressing the bacterial culprit in H. pylori infections or mitigating excessive acid production, each medication plays a defined role in unraveling the complexities of your condition.

3. BALANCING SYMPTOM RELIEF AND LONG-TERM WELLNESS:

Beyond symptom relief, medications are chosen to promote long-term wellness. This distinctive approach seeks not only to alleviate immediate discomfort but also to lay the groundwork for sustained health, fostering a balance between immediate relief and enduring well-being.

4. MONITORING AND ADJUSTING TREATMENT PLANS:

The treatment journey unfolds dynamically, with healthcare professionals monitoring the effects of medications closely.

Regular assessments allow for adjustments in treatment plans, ensuring that interventions evolve in tandem with your response to medications, fostering an adaptive and responsive healing trajectory.

5. EMPOWERING THROUGH EDUCATION:

A vital aspect of the treatment journey involves empowering you with knowledge. Understanding the mechanisms and potential side effects of medications equips you to actively engage in your well-being. This shared knowledge forms the basis for informed decisions and a collaborative approach to treatment.

6. PERSONALIZED APPROACHES TO MINIMIZE SIDE EFFECTS:

Recognizing the individuality of health responses, healthcare professionals strive to minimize side effects by tailoring medication choices. This personalized approach acknowledges your unique sensitivities and preferences, enhancing the overall treatment experience.

In this distinctive tapestry of treatment, medications emerge not just as remedies but as integral threads woven into the fabric of your healing journey. The impact of each medication is unique, contributing to a narrative of resilience, adaptation, and a pursuit of enduring wellness.

MANAGEMENT

ERADICATION STRATEGIES

Current guidelines recommend H. pylori eradication therapy for all patients with duodenal and gastric ulcers when the bacterium is present. However, the decision for eradication therapy in patients with incidental H. pylori infection and no ulcers remains a subject of controversy.

The recent surge in the prevalence of GORD and adenocarcinoma of the lower esophagus has been observed without a clear explanation, leading to speculations about its potential association with H. pylori eradication. While this link is not disproven, its likelihood remains uncertain.

In developed nations, standard eradication therapies boast a success rate of approximately 90%, with re-infection being a rare occurrence (1%). However, in developing countries, where metronidazole resistance is high and treatment compliance may be challenging, eradication failure is more common.

Despite the array of available eradication regimens, certain considerations must be factored in:

- **Emphasis on Good Compliance:**

Successful outcomes hinge on patient compliance, making it crucial to tailor regimens that align with individual lifestyles and preferences.

- **Addressing Antibiotic Resistance Challenges:**

Resistance to metronidazole and clarithromycin is noteworthy, especially in specific populations. The resistance to clarithromycin has doubled in Europe over the past decade.

Navigating Side Effects and Acceptance:

- The use of oral metronidazole and bismuth chelate is not without challenges, with metronidazole often causing side effects and bismuth chelate being regarded as unpleasant, even in tablet form.

Key agents in eradication regimens include metronidazole, clarithromycin, amoxicillin, tetracycline, and bismuth. Notably, resistance to amoxicillin (1–2%) and tetracycline (<1%) remains low, except in regions where these antibiotics are available without prescription, leading to potential higher resistance rates.

In cases of treatment failure with standard regimens, alternative options such as quinolones (e.g., ciprofloxacin), furazolidone, and rifabutin are employed as 'rescue therapy.' However, these drugs are not effective in isolation, and eradication regimens typically involve a combination of two antibiotics along with potent acid suppression, often in the form of a proton pump inhibitor (PPI).

Bismuth-containing quadruple therapy is now recommended as first-line treatment, especially in regions with escalating clarithromycin resistance. The conventional clarithromycin-based triple therapy has taken a backseat in areas where resistance rates are high. This evolving landscape underscores the importance of adapting eradication strategies to both local resistance patterns and individual patient needs.

ILLUSTRATIVE TREATMENT PLANS

REGIMEN VARIATIONS:

Diverse treatment plans exist, such as Omeprazole 20 mg combined with clarithromycin 500 mg and amoxicillin 1g, both administered twice daily. Another option involves Omeprazole 20 mg paired with metronidazole 400 mg and clarithromycin 500 mg, also taken twice daily. These regimens are typically administered for 7 or 14 days, with the latter associated with enhanced eradication rates despite potential heightened side effects impacting ccompliance.

- ADAPTING TO ERADICATION CHALLENGES:

In instances of eradication failure or regions with clarithromycin resistance, a comprehensive approach includes bismuth chelate (120 mg four times daily), metronidazole (400 mg three times daily), tetracycline (500 mg four times daily), and a PPI (20–40 mg twice daily) over 14 days. Sequential therapy, involving 5 days of PPI and amoxicillin followed by a 5-day period of PPI with clarithromycin and tinidazole, is also employed in such cases. The surge in clarithromycin resistance has led to the adoption of this quadruple therapy as an initial treatment choice.

- POST-THERAPY ASSESSMENT:

Prolonged PPI therapy following a 7-day triple therapy with PP as a base is generally unnecessary for ulcer healing in most H. pylori-infected patients. Assessment of treatment effectiveness for uncomplicated duodenal ulcers is primarily symptomatic. Persistent symptoms warrant breath or stool testing to verify eradication (off PPI therapy).

- MONITORING HIGH-RISK CASES:

Patients at risk of bleeding or those with complications like hemorrhage or perforation should undergo a 13C-urea breath test or stool test for H. pylori six weeks post-treatment completion to ensure successful eradication.

Consideration of long-term PPIs may be essential in scenarios where a rebleed could be potentially fatal.

- HOLISTIC APPROACHES:

Encouraging smoking cessation is a vital aspect of general measures, recognizing its impact on slowing mucosal healing. Routine re-endoscopy at 6 weeks for patients with gastric ulcers is advised to confirm mucosal healing and rule out underlying gastric cancer. Repeat biopsies may be necessary to ensure a comprehensive evaluation.

In crafting these unique treatment strategies, the emphasis lies not only on eradication efficacy but also on tailoring approaches to individual patient needs and responding dynamically to evolving challenges in H. pylori management.

The complications of peptic ulcers may include:

1. Bleeding:

Ulcers can cause bleeding, leading to symptoms such as hematemesis (vomiting blood) or melena (dark, tarry stools).

2. Perforation:

In severe cases, ulcers may penetrate through the wall of the stomach or duodenum, causing a perforation. This can result in sudden and intense abdominal pain.

3. Gastric Outlet Obstruction:

Scarring from chronic ulcers may obstruct the passage of food from the stomach to the small intestine, causing symptoms like persistent vomiting and weight loss.

4. Peritonitis:

If an ulcer perforates and spills its contents into the abdominal cavity, it can lead to peritonitis, causing severe abdominal pain and tenderness.

5. Penetration into Adjacent Organs:

Ulcers may penetrate nearby organs, such as the liver or pancreas, leading to complications specific to those organs.

6. Gastrointestinal Strictures:

Long-term inflammation and scarring can lead to the formation of strictures, narrowing the gastrointestinal tract and causing difficulties in food passage.

7. Increased Risk of Gastric Cancer:

Chronic H. pylori infection and long-standing peptic ulcers may elevate the risk of developing gastric cancer, although this is a relatively rare complication.

It's important to note that not all individuals with peptic ulcers will experience complications, and timely medical intervention can often prevent or manage these serious outcomes.

LIFESTYLE ADJUSTMENTS TO EFFECTIVELY MANAGE PEPTIC ULCERS

Successfully managing peptic ulcers involves not only medical interventions but also adopting lifestyle changes that promote healing and reduce the risk of complications. These modifications contribute to a holistic approach, fostering a supportive environment for ulcer recovery.

1. DIETARY MODIFICATIONS:

Avoid trigger foods: Steering clear of foods that can exacerbate ulcer symptoms, such as spicy, acidic, or highly caffeinated items, can significantly contribute to symptom relief.

Frequent, Small Meals: Opting for smaller, more frequent meals throughout the day rather than three large meals helps minimize stomach acid production and promote digestion without overloading the system.

2. SMOKING CESSATION:

Quitting smoking is crucial in ulcer management, as smoking has been linked to delayed mucosal healing. Breaking this habit accelerates the healing process.

3. LIMITING ALCOHOL CONSUMPTION:

Moderating alcohol intake is advisable, as excessive alcohol consumption can irritate the stomach lining and potentially impede the healing of peptic ulcers.

4. STRESS REDUCTION TECHNIQUES:

Engaging in stress-reducing activities, such as meditation, deep breathing exercises, or yoga, can be beneficial. Stress management plays a role in preventing the exacerbation of ulcer symptoms.

5. HYDRATION:

Staying well-hydrated supports overall digestive health and aids in mucosal healing. Opting for water or non-caffeinated herbal teas is particularly advisable.

6. MEDICATION ADHERENCE:

Adhering to prescribed medications, such as proton pump inhibitors (PPIs) or antibiotics for H. pylori eradication, is crucial for successful ulcer treatment. Patients should follow their prescribed dosage and complete the full course of medications.

7. REGULAR EXERCISE:

Engaging in regular, moderate exercise contributes to overall well-being and may help manage stress. However, individuals with peptic ulcers should consult their healthcare provider to determine the most suitable exercise routine.

8. APPROPRIATE NSAID USE:

If nonsteroidal anti-inflammatory drugs (NSAIDs) are deemed necessary, using them cautiously and under medical supervision is essential. Some NSAIDs can contribute to ulcer formation or exacerbate existing ulcers.

9. REGULAR CHECK-UPS AND MONITORING:

Routine follow-up appointments with healthcare providers allow for the assessment of ulcer healing progress and adjustments to the treatment plan, if necessary.

10. MAINTAINING A HEALTHY WEIGHT:

Achieving and maintaining a healthy weight through a balanced diet and regular exercise is beneficial for overall health and may positively impact ulcer management.

These lifestyle changes, when integrated into a comprehensive treatment plan, contribute to an environment conducive to ulcer healing and long-term well-being. Individuals with peptic ulcers should collaborate closely with healthcare professionals to tailor these adjustments to their specific needs and circumstances.

8

DIET AND NUTRITION GUIDANCE: NOURISHING CHOICES FOR PEPTIC ULCER MANAGEMENT

Crafting a dietary approach tailored to support peptic ulcer management involves a thoughtful selection of foods that promote healing while avoiding those that may exacerbate symptoms. Here's a guide to foods to include and those to avoid:

FOODS TO INCLUDE:

1. High-Fiber Options:

Incorporate whole grains, fruits, vegetables, and legumes rich in fiber. These foods contribute to digestive health and may help regulate bowel movements.

2. Lean proteins:

Choose low-fat protein options such as skinless poultry, fish, tofu, and legumes. Protein is essential for tissue repair and overall health.

3. Probiotic-rich foods:

Include yogurt with live cultures, kefir, and other fermented foods to promote a healthy balance of gut bacteria. Probiotics may support digestive health.

4. Healthy fats:

Select sources of beneficial fats like avocados, olive oil, and fatty fish such as salmon. These fats can provide essential nutrients without contributing to excess stomach acid.

5. Low-Acidity Fruits:

Opt for low-acidity fruits like bananas, melons, and pears. These are less likely to irritate the stomach lining.

6. Non-Citrus Vegetables:

Embrace non-citrus vegetables, such as leafy greens, carrots, and broccoli, which provide vitamins and minerals without excess acidity.

7. Complex Carbohydrates:

Prioritize complex carbohydrates like brown rice, quinoa, and sweet potatoes. These can provide sustained energy without causing spikes in stomach acid.

8. Herbal Teas:

Choose non-caffeinated herbal teas, such as chamomile or ginger tea. These can be soothing to the digestive system.

FOODS TO AVOID:

1. Spicy foods:

Limit or avoid spicy foods, as they can irritate the stomach lining and exacerbate ulcer symptoms.

2. High-Acidity Fruits:

Steer clear of highly acidic fruits like oranges, tomatoes, and citrus juices, which can increase stomach acid.

3. **Caffeine:**

Reduce or eliminate caffeinated beverages, as caffeine can stimulate acid production. This includes coffee, tea, and certain sodas.

4. **Alcohol:**

Limit alcohol intake, as it can irritate the stomach lining and potentially interfere with the healing process.

5. **Fried and Fatty Foods:**

Avoid fried and fatty foods, as they can delay gastric emptying and contribute to increased acid production.

6. **Processed and Spicy Meats:**

Minimize processed meats and spicy preparations, as they may be harsh on the stomach.

7. **Mint and peppermint:**

Steer clear of mint and peppermint, as they can relax the lower esophageal sphincter, potentially leading to increased acid reflux.

8. **Carbonated Beverages:**

Limit carbonated beverages, as they can contribute to bloating and may exacerbate symptoms.

Individual responses to foods can vary, so it's essential to observe how specific items impact personal comfort and adjust the diet accordingly. Consulting with healthcare professionals or a registered dietitian can provide personalized guidance tailored to individual needs and preferences.

WHICH FOODS SUPPORT STOMACH ULCER MANAGEMENT?

As the discovery of the role of H. pylori bacteria in ulcer development unfolds, researchers are investigating foods that may aid in combating this infection. Alongside the antibiotics and acid-blocking medications prescribed by your doctor, incorporating these foods into your diet might offer additional support against ulcer-causing bacteria:

- Cauliflower
- Cabbage
- Radishes
- Apples
- Berries (blueberries, raspberries, blackberries, strawberries, cherries)
- Bell peppers
- Carrots
- Broccoli
- Leafy greens (kale, spinach)
- Probiotic-rich foods (yogurt, kefir, miso, sauerkraut, kombucha)
- Olive oil and other plant-based oils
- Honey
- Garlic
- Decaffeinated green tea
- Licorice
- Turmeric

WHY ARE THEY BENEFICIAL?

If your stomach ulcer stems from an H. pylori infection, foods rich in antioxidants may play a beneficial role. These foods can potentially activate your immune system, aiding in the fight against infection and protecting against stomach cancer. Notable examples include:

Antioxidant-Packed Foods: Blueberries, cherries, and bell peppers.

Leafy greens: kale and spinach, containing calcium and B vitamins.

Sulforaphane-rich Broccoli exhibits anti-H. pylori activity.

Olive Oil: Fatty acids may contribute to H. pylori treatment.

Probiotic Foods: Miso, sauerkraut, and kimchi may prevent reinfection.

Turmeric: is currently under study as a potential treatment for ulcers.

Garlic, decaffeinated green tea, and licorice are included for their potential benefits.

Consider Supplements:

For those undergoing antibiotic treatment for a stomach ulcer, integrating a probiotic supplement into your diet plan may be beneficial. This can alleviate antibiotic-associated symptoms and enhance antibiotic effectiveness. Lactobacillus, Bifidobacterium, and Saccharomyces supplements have shown promise in H. pylori ulcer cases.

Deglycyrrhizinated licorice (taken one hour before meals) and curcumin extracts are being explored in ulcer research due to their potential effectiveness against H. pylori.

NAVIGATING FOODS TO AVOID:

For individuals dealing with both ulcers and acid reflux, certain foods that relax the lower esophageal sphincter should be approached with caution. Understanding your body's response to specific foods is crucial to tailoring a diet that promotes healing while minimizing discomfort.

A loosened lower esophageal sphincter (LES) facilitates the regurgitation of acid into the esophagus, leading to symptoms like heartburn, indigestion, and discomfort.

Consuming certain foods can potentially exacerbate acid reflux. These include:

- Coffee
- Chocolate
- Spicy dishes
- Alcoholic beverages
- Acidic foods, such as citrus and tomatoes
- Caffeine

Additionally, overindulgence and eating close to bedtime, within two to three hours before sleep, might further intensify symptoms of reflux.

INNOVATIVE MEAL PLANNING STRATEGIES FOR PEPTIC ULCER WELL-BEING

Crafting a meal plan for individuals managing peptic ulcers involves a blend of creativity and nutritional wisdom. This unique approach goes beyond conventional guidelines, tailoring dietary choices to enhance healing and provide a culinary experience that promotes overall well-being.

1. Balanced Flavor Profiles:

Infuse meals with a variety of herbs and spices to enhance flavor without relying on excessive salt or irritants. Experiment with herbs like basil, oregano, and turmeric for both taste and potential anti-inflammatory benefits.

2. Colorful Culinary Palette:

Embrace a vibrant array of fruits and vegetables to not only provide essential nutrients but also create visually appealing and appetizing dishes. A colorful plate signifies a diverse range of beneficial compounds.

3. Texture Exploration:

Explore textures to add interest and satisfaction to meals. Incorporate crunchy elements like nuts or seeds into salads or opt for smooth and soothing textures in soups and purees.

4. Hydration Variety:

Diversify hydration options beyond plain water. Experiment with infused waters, herbal teas, or diluted fruit juices for a refreshing twist. Maintaining proper hydration is essential for digestive well-being.

5. Mindful Meal Timing:

Integrate mindful eating practices by focusing on the sensory experience of each meal. Pay attention to flavors, textures, and the satisfaction of nourishing your body.

6. Adventurous Alternatives:

Venture into alternative grains like quinoa, farro, or barley to add nutritional richness and a delightful change to the usual starch options.

7. Protein Playfulness:

Infuse creativity into protein sources. Explore plant-based proteins like lentils or chickpeas alongside lean meats or fish. This not only broadens nutritional intake but also introduces exciting culinary possibilities.

8. Prebiotic and Probiotic Prowess:

Integrate prebiotic-rich foods like garlic, onions, and leeks to support a healthy gut environment. Probiotic-rich options such as yogurt or fermented foods contribute to digestive balance.

9. Collaborative Cooking:

Engage in collaborative meal planning and preparation. Involving friends or family in the process can make mealtime a shared experience, fostering a positive and supportive atmosphere.

10. Intuitive Eating Empowerment:

Encourage intuitive eating by recognizing and respecting individual hunger and fullness cues. This personalized approach promotes a healthy relationship with food.

By infusing meal planning with innovation and a sense of exploration, individuals managing peptic ulcers can enjoy a diverse, nourishing, and satisfying culinary experience. This approach not only supports physical well-being but also enhances the pleasure derived from each dining occasion.

9

NURTURING EMOTIONAL RESILIENCE: STRATEGIES FOR MANAGING STRESS AND ANXIETY

Cultivating emotional and mental well-being is a pivotal aspect of comprehensive health, especially for individuals navigating the challenges of peptic ulcers. Here, we explore innovative and personalized approaches to cope with stress and anxiety, fostering a resilient mindset.

1. MINDFUL BREATHING BREAKS:

Integrate brief, mindful breathing exercises into your daily routine. A few minutes of focused, deep breathing can provide a moment of calm amidst the demands of the day, promoting emotional equilibrium.

2. EXPRESSIVE WRITING JOURNEY:

Embark on an expressive writing journey to articulate and process emotions. Journaling offers a therapeutic outlet, allowing you to explore and understand the intricate layers of your feelings.

3. ARTISTIC EXPLORATION:

Engage in creative endeavors such as drawing, painting, or crafting. Artistic expression serves as a unique channel to channel emotions and immerse oneself in a positive and absorbing activity.

4. HOLISTIC STRESS-REDUCING PRACTICES:

Explore holistic practices like yoga, tai chi, or meditation. These practices not only enhance physical well-being but also provide a holistic approach to stress management, harmonizing mind and body.

5. PERSONALIZED RELAXATION PLAYLISTS:

Curate playlists of music or sounds that resonate with tranquility. Listening to personalized relaxation playlists can serve as an auditory escape, transporting you to a mental space of calm.

6. CONNECTIVE SOCIAL SUPPORT:

Cultivate relationships with understanding friends, family, or supportive communities. Sharing experiences and feelings with others who understand can alleviate the emotional burden and provide a sense of belonging.

7. MINDFULNESS IN EATING:

Practice mindfulness during meals by savoring each bite. Creating a mindful eating environment not only aids digestion but also encourages a moment of reprieve from daily stressors.

8. NATURE IMMERSION:

Immerse yourself in nature, even if it's just for a short walk in a nearby park. Nature has a soothing effect on the mind and can serve as a grounding experience amidst the hustle of daily life.

9. GRATITUDE RITUALS:

Establish daily gratitude rituals by reflecting on positive aspects of your life. Focusing on gratitude can shift your mindset and enhance your overall emotional well-being.

10. PROFESSIONAL SUPPORT EXPLORATION:

Consider exploring professional support through therapy or counseling. Talking to a mental health professional provides a safe space to navigate emotions and develop coping strategies tailored to your unique needs.

By embracing these personalized strategies, individuals can build emotional resilience, effectively cope with stress and anxiety, and create a foundation for enduring mental well-being while managing the challenges associated with peptic ulcers.

BUILDING A ROBUST SUPPORT NETWORK FOR INDIVIDUALS WITH PEPTIC ULCERS

Navigating the journey of managing peptic ulcers is not a solitary endeavor. Establishing a strong support system is paramount for both emotional well-being and practical assistance. Here's a guide to crafting a robust support network:

1. FAMILY AND FRIENDS:

Lean on the understanding and care of family members and friends. Share your experiences, concerns, and triumphs with those close to you. Their support can provide emotional solace and encouragement.

2. PATIENT SUPPORT GROUPS:

Joining patient support groups, either in person or online, offers a valuable opportunity to connect with individuals facing similar challenges. Sharing insights, strategies, and encouragement within these communities fosters a sense of belonging and understanding.

3. HEALTHCARE PROFESSIONALS:

Forge a collaborative partnership with your healthcare team. Regular communication with your doctors, nurses, and dietitians ensures that you stay informed about your condition and receive tailored guidance for managing peptic ulcers.

4. MENTAL HEALTH PROFESSIONALS:

Consider seeking support from mental health professionals, such as counselors or therapists. Dealing with a chronic condition can be emotionally taxing, and professional guidance can provide coping strategies and emotional resilience.

5. WORKPLACE ALLIES:

Communicate with your workplace about your condition, especially if it affects your daily routine. Colleagues and supervisors can offer support and reasonable accommodations, creating a conducive environment for optimal well-being.

6. HOLISTIC PRACTITIONERS:

Explore complementary and alternative practitioners, such as nutritionists, acupuncturists, or holistic therapists. Integrating holistic approaches alongside conventional medical care can enhance overall well-being.

7. EDUCATIONAL RESOURCES:

Stay informed about your condition through reputable educational resources. Understanding the nuances of peptic ulcers empowers you to actively participate in your care and make informed decisions.

8. SPOUSAL OR PARTNER SUPPORT:

If applicable, foster open communication with your spouse or partner. Their understanding and support are crucial in navigating both the practical and emotional aspects of managing peptic ulcers

9. FINANCIAL ADVISORS:

If financial concerns arise due to medical expenses or changes in work capacity, consult financial advisors who specialize in healthcare planning.

Understanding your options can alleviate the stress associated with financial uncertainties.

10. COMMUNITY ENGAGEMENT:

Engage with your local community or online forums dedicated to health and wellness. Connecting with a broader community provides diverse perspectives and a sense of solidarity in your journey.

Remember, building a support system is a dynamic process that evolves as your needs change. Regularly assess your support network and communicate openly with those involved. By weaving together these various strands of support, individuals with peptic ulcers can fortify their resilience and face the challenges ahead with collective strength.

10

PREVENTION STRATEGIES: LIFESTYLE MODIFICATIONS

Preventing peptic ulcers involves crafting a personalized strategy that transcends conventional wisdom. Explore these unique lifestyle modifications to forge a path toward optimal well-being:

1. CULINARY ALCHEMY:

Embrace the art of culinary alchemy by experimenting with anti-inflammatory herbs and spices. Incorporate turmeric, ginger, and cinnamon into your meals, not only for their rich flavors but also for their potential healing properties.

2. MINDFUL NUTRIENT SYNERGY:

Curate meals that promote nutrient synergy. Pairing vitamin C-rich foods with iron sources enhances iron absorption, potentially supporting mucosal healing. Explore combinations like bell peppers with lean poultry for a synergistic nutrient boost.

3. SLEEP SANCTUARIES:

Transform your sleep environment into a sanctuary for restorative rest. Experiment with calming aromatherapy, comfortable bedding, and sleep hygiene practices to ensure quality sleep—a cornerstone of overall well-being.

4. JOYFUL PHYSICAL ACTIVITY:

Infuse joy into your physical activity routine. Whether it's dancing, hiking, or trying a new fitness class, finding activities that bring delight not only promotes physical health but also contributes to stress reduction.

5. TECH-FACILITATED MINDFULNESS:

harness technology for mindfulness. Explore meditation and relaxation apps that guide you through moments of tranquility, fostering emotional resilience, and mitigating stress—a key component in ulcer prevention.

6. EPICUREAN EXPLORATION:

Embark on an epicurean journey by discovering unconventional, ulcer-friendly recipes. Explore the world of plant-based gastronomy, experimenting with nutrient-rich, inflammation-soothing ingredients for culinary excitement.

7. DIGITAL DETOX RETREATS:

Schedule regular digital detox retreats to unplug from the constant digital buzz. Engaging in screen-free periods promotes mental clarity and allows you to reconnect with activities that bring joy and relaxation.

8. HERBAL INFUSIONS:

Embrace the world of herbal infusions. Beyond traditional teas, explore infusions with chamomile, licorice, and marshmallow root. These botanical allies may contribute to digestive comfort and mucosal support.

9. NATURE'S THERAPY:

Immerse yourself in nature's therapy. Regularly spend time outdoors, whether it's a stroll in a nearby park or a weekend hiking adventure. Nature has a profound impact on mental well-being and can be a powerful preventative ally.

10. EXPRESSIVE ARTS INTEGRATION:

Integrate expressive arts into your routine. Whether it's doodling, playing an instrument, or trying your hand at poetry, creative expression serves as an outlet for emotions and contributes to holistic well-being.

Remember, prevention is not a one-size-fits-all endeavor. These lifestyle modifications are a canvas for you to paint a unique and vibrant picture of prevention—one that aligns with your preferences, fosters joy, and propels you toward enduring well-being.

LONG-TERM HEALTH MASTERY: SUSTAINING WELLNESS BEYOND PEPTIC ULCERS

The journey to managing peptic ulcers extends far beyond immediate treatment. Long-term health maintenance becomes a focal point, intertwining medical insights with lifestyle choices for enduring well-being:

1. DYNAMIC NUTRITIONAL VIGILANCE:

Cultivate an ever-evolving awareness of nutritional needs. Regularly reassess your dietary choices, emphasizing a balance of nutrient-dense foods. Collaborate with a nutritionist to fine-tune your dietary plan as your health evolves.

2. HOLISTIC FITNESS FUSION:

Foster a holistic approach to fitness by blending various forms of exercise. Incorporate strength training, flexibility exercises, and cardiovascular activities into your routine. Regularly revisit and adjust your fitness regimen to match your evolving health goals.

3. MIND-BODY SYNERGY PRACTICES:

Integrate mind-body synergy practices into your daily life. Explore yoga, tai chi, or mindfulness meditation to establish a resilient connection between mental and physical well-being. These practices lay a foundation for stress management and holistic health.

4. CONSISTENT MEDICAL CHECKPOINTS:

Maintain consistent medical check-ins with your healthcare team. Regular appointments ensure ongoing monitoring of your health status and allow for prompt adjustments to your treatment plan if needed.

5. STRATEGIC STRESS RESPONSE:

Develop personalized strategies for stress response. Understand your unique stressors and cultivate coping mechanisms that align with your values. This proactive approach supports mental resilience, a key element in sustaining long-term health.

6. SLEEP QUALITY OPTIMIZATION:

Prioritize and optimize sleep quality. Establish a consistent sleep routine, create a comfortable sleep environment, and address any sleep-related issues promptly. Quality sleep contributes significantly to overall health maintenance.

7. CONTINUOUS LEARNING PATH:

Embrace a continuous learning path regarding your health condition. Stay informed about advancements in peptic ulcer research, treatment options, and lifestyle recommendations. Knowledge empowers you to actively participate in your long-term well-being.

8. COMMUNITY CONNECTION CULTIVATION:

Cultivate connections within your community. Engage in activities that foster a sense of belonging and mutual support. Social connections contribute to emotional well-being, forming a crucial aspect of long-term health.

9. ADAPTIVE RESILIENCE BUILDING:

Foster adaptive resilience by embracing change and adapting to evolving health circumstances. Life is dynamic, and your approach to well-being should be flexible, allowing you to navigate challenges with resilience and optimism.

10. JOYFUL LIVING PURSUIT:

Make the pursuit of joy an integral part of your life. Engage in activities that bring fulfillment, happiness, and a sense of purpose. The pursuit of joy not only enhances mental well-being but also contributes to a holistic and gratifying existence.

Long-term health maintenance is a multifaceted journey that requires a proactive and adaptive mindset. By intertwining medical guidance with lifestyle choices, you can sculpt a future characterized by sustained well-being beyond the challenges of peptic ulcers.

11

FREQUENTLY ASKED QUESTIONS ON PEPTIC ULCERS

1. WHAT ARE PEPTIC ULCERS, AND HOW DO THEY DEVELOP?

Peptic ulcers are open sores that develop on the inner lining of the stomach, upper small intestine, or esophagus. They often result from the erosion caused by stomach acid, H. pylori infection, or the use of nonsteroidal anti-inflammatory drugs (NSAIDs).

2. WHAT SYMPTOMS INDICATE THE PRESENCE OF PEPTIC ULCERS?

Common symptoms include burning stomach pain, bloating, nausea, vomiting, and a feeling of fullness. Severe cases can lead to complications such as bleeding or perforation.

3. HOW IS H. PYLORI INFECTION DIAGNOSED?

Diagnosis typically involves a breath test, blood test, stool test, or endoscopy to detect the presence of Helicobacter pylori bacteria. Treatment for H. pylori often involves a combination of antibiotics and acid-reducing medications.

4. CAN PEPTIC ULCERS BE PREVENTED?

Adopting a healthy lifestyle, avoiding NSAIDs when possible, managing stress, and treating H. pylori infections promptly can contribute to ulcer prevention. Personalized lifestyle modifications play a crucial role in long-term prevention.

5. WHAT DIETARY CHANGES CAN HELP MANAGE PEPTIC ULCERS?

Focus on a well-balanced diet rich in fruits, vegetables, lean proteins, and whole grains. Avoiding spicy foods, caffeine, and alcohol while embracing anti-inflammatory choices can support ulcer management.

6. ARE PEPTIC ULCERS LINKED TO STRESS?

While stress doesn't directly cause ulcers, it can exacerbate symptoms and slow the healing process. Stress management techniques, such as mindfulness and relaxation exercises, are beneficial for overall well-being.

7. HOW LONG DOES IT TAKE FOR PEPTIC ULCERS TO HEAL?

The healing duration varies based on factors such as the underlying cause, severity, and treatment adherence. With proper care, many ulcers heal within a few weeks, but follow-up appointments are crucial for monitoring progress.

8. IS SURGERY ALWAYS REQUIRED FOR PEPTIC ULCERS?

Surgery is rarely the first-line treatment for peptic ulcers. Medications, lifestyle changes, and addressing the underlying causes are often effective. Surgery may be considered for complications like bleeding or perforation.

9. CAN PEPTIC ULCERS RECUR?

Yes, peptic ulcers can recur. Managing underlying causes, adopting a healthy lifestyle, and staying vigilant about symptoms are essential for preventing recurrence.

10. HOW CAN I SUPPORT SOMEONE WITH PEPTIC ULCERS?

Offer empathy, encourage adherence to medical advice, and participate in healthy lifestyle practices together. Understanding the challenges they face and providing emotional support contribute significantly to their well-being.

These answers provide a foundation for understanding and managing peptic ulcers. However, individual cases may vary, and consulting with healthcare professionals remains paramount for personalized guidance.

DISPELLING MYTHS: UNRAVELING COMMON MISCONCEPTIONS ABOUT PEPTIC ULCERS

Myth 1: SPICY FOODS CAUSE PEPTIC ULCERS

Reality: Spicy foods might exacerbate symptoms but don't directly cause ulcers. The primary culprits are H. pylori infection, NSAID use, and excessive stomach acid.

Myth 2: ONLY STRESS LEADS TO PEPTIC ULCERS

Reality: Stress contributes to symptom aggravation, but it's not a direct cause. H. pylori infection and NSAID use play more significant roles in ulcer development.

Myth 3: ULCERS ALWAYS CAUSE PAIN

Reality: Ulcers can be asymptomatic or present with subtle symptoms. Some individuals may not experience pain, making regular check-ups crucial for detection.

Myth 4: MILK SOOTHES ULCER PAIN

Reality: While milk might temporarily alleviate symptoms, it doesn't aid in ulcer healing. In some cases, dairy can stimulate acid production, worsening discomfort.

Myth 5: PEPTIC ULCERS ARE ONLY IN THE STOMACH

Reality: Ulcers can develop in the stomach, small intestine, or esophagus. Understanding the location is vital for effective treatment.

Myth 6: ULCERS MEAN A STRICT NO TO SPICY FOOD FOREVER

Reality: Moderation is key. While excessive spice may irritate, enjoying well-tolerated amounts is acceptable for many individuals.

Myth 7: ANTACIDS CURE PEPTIC ULCERS

Reality: Antacids offer symptom relief but don't cure ulcers. Medical treatments targeting H. pylori or reducing acid production are essential for healing.

Myth 8: ONLY OLDER ADULTS GET PEPTIC ULCERS

Reality: Ulcers can affect individuals of any age. Factors like H. pylori infection and NSAID use impact a broad demographic.

Myth 9: PEPTIC ULCERS ALWAYS REQUIRE SURGERY

Reality: Surgery is rare and usually reserved for severe complications. Medications, lifestyle changes, and endoscopic treatments are often effective.

Myth 10: ONCE HEALED, PEPTIC ULCERS WON'T RECUR

Reality: Recurrence is possible. Managing underlying causes, adhering to treatment plans, and adopting a healthy lifestyle are crucial for prevention.

By dispelling these myths, we aim to foster an accurate understanding and empower individuals to make informed decisions about peptic ulcer prevention and management. Always consult healthcare professionals for personalized advice.

CONCLUSION

As we near the end of "What Your Doctor May Not Tell You About Peptic Ulcers," it is more than simply the conclusion of a book. It is a turning point in your own journey, one that has evolved through the complexities of learning, growing, and being an active participant.

Peptic ulcer research has been more than just that—a lively conversation, an open exchange of ideas on this health problem that has yet to have its answers revealed. Recognizing that your path is a tapestry of tales, perseverance, and personal achievements, we have walked you through the clinical intricacies, debunked falsehoods, and given you tools to empower yourself.

This book isn't ending; it's inviting you to take the lessons learned with you into the rest of your life. I pray that you go on with confidence, knowing that knowledge is your greatest asset in the fight for health.

This is only the beginning; your path will continue to change and progress. Even after this book's pages close, the story of your life, woven with the wisdom you've gained from reading it, will go on. This book serves as a foundation for your continued empowerment and knowledge of peptic ulcers, whether you are just starting out or have reached major milestones along the way.

By the time you reach the end of this book, I hope you've gained the knowledge and insight to make well-informed decisions, the courage to persevere through tough times, and the constant reminder that your story is a product of your own decisions, strengths, and developing knowledge of health.

Thank you for being a part of this journey. May your future be blessed with health, resilience, and a great feeling of well-being.